ACUPUNCTURE THERAPY FOR BEGINNERS

Unlocking The Power Of Traditional Chinese Medicine For Pain Relief, Stress Reduction, And Overall Well-Being- Your Key To Balancing Energy And Alleviating Ailments

DR. ARIYA REYNA

CONTENTS

DISCLIAMER

This book is intended for informational purposes only and is not a substitute for professional medical advice, diagnosis, or treatment. The information provided in this book is based on the author's research and personal experiences and is not meant to replace the advice of healthcare professionals.

Readers are encouraged to consult with their healthcare providers before beginning any new exercise, wellness, or health program.

The author and publisher of this book are not responsible for any specific health or allergy needs that may require medical supervision and are not liable for any damages or negative consequences from any treatment, action, application, or preparation, to any person reading or following the information in this book.

The content of this book is not intended to be a substitute for professional medical advice, diagnosis, or treatment. Always seek the advice of your physician or other qualified health provider with any questions you may have regarding a medical condition.

The author and publisher disclaim responsibility for any adverse effects that may result from the use or application of the information contained in this book.

References to specific products, services, or organizations do not imply endorsement or recommendation by the author or the publisher.

The inclusion of such references is for illustrative purposes only. Thank you for reading and respecting the terms outlined in this disclaimer.

CHAPTER ONE

Acupuncture Fundamentals

Acupuncture is a traditional Chinese treatment that has acquired a worldwide reputation for its effectiveness in treating a variety of medical ailments. Acupuncture, which has its roots in ancient Chinese medicine, involves inserting small needles into particular places on the body to increase energy flow and restore balance. While the technique has gained popularity across the world, its cultural origins and values are firmly rooted in the rich tapestry of Chinese medicinal traditions.

Acupuncture's underlying idea is based on the concept of Qi (pronounced "chee"), an important life energy that travels through the body along paths known as meridians. A healthy flow of Qi is understood to be essential for optimum health, and interruptions in this flow are thought to cause a variety of diseases. Acupuncture seeks to restore the balanced flow of Qi, therefore enhancing general well-being.

Acupuncture's Historical Foundations

Acupuncture has a long history that dates back thousands of years and is intricately entwined with the old Chinese medical system. The oldest known references to acupuncture may be found in ancient manuscripts dating back to the 2nd century BCE, such as the Huangdi Neijing (Yellow Emperor's Inner Canon). This introductory work discusses the fundamentals of traditional Chinese medicine (TCM) and delves into the philosophy and procedures of acupuncture.

According to historical sources, acupuncture evolved over the ages as a result of Chinese physicians' observations and experiences. Taoist philosophy, which stressed the balance of opposing forces in nature and the body, impacted the creation of acupuncture. Acupuncture gradually became an essential component of TCM, a holistic approach to treatment that recognizes the interdependence of the body, mind, and spirit.

Traditional Chinese Medicine Principles

Traditional Chinese Medicine (TCM), a holistic approach that views the body as a complex network of interrelated systems, is profoundly anchored in the concepts of acupuncture. TCM acknowledges the dynamic balance of opposing forces like as Yin and Yang, as well as the movement of vital energy or Qi throughout the body. When these energies are out of balance or there is a barrier in the passage of Qi, sickness can occur.

The body is viewed as a microcosm of the natural world in TCM, and the Yin and Yang principles represent the duality essence of life. Yin denotes darkness, calm, and receptivity, whereas Yang represents light, activity, and warmth. Acupuncture is one of the instruments used to restore equilibrium between these conflicting forces, and it is regarded as a state of balance between these opposing forces.

Acupoints And Meridians

The meridians, or energy lines that cross the body and enable the passage of Qi, are central to acupuncture philosophy. These meridians are related to certain organs and functions, and disturbances in their flow are thought to be linked to a variety of health problems. There are 12 basic meridians, each linked with a distinct organ, and eight exceptional meridians, which play an important role in managing the general balance of the body.

Acupoints, also known as acupuncture points, are precise points along the meridians that may be used to access and alter the flow of Qi. These locations are frequently found in places where energy is supposed to be easily impacted.

Acupoint stimulation via needle insertion, pressure, or other procedures is intended to rectify imbalances in the flow of Qi and promote the body's natural healing processes.

Acupuncture Methods

Acupuncture procedures vary, and practitioners may use a variety of techniques depending on the individual's condition and the intended therapeutic effect. The most popular approach involves inserting fine, sterile needles into acupoints, which is often painless and accompanied by a distinct feeling known as "de qi," which is commonly described as a tingling or dull ache and is said to indicate that the Qi has been activated.

Other treatments, in addition to standard needle acupuncture, include:

1. Electroacupuncture is a technique that includes connecting electrodes to acupuncture needles to provide a mild electrical current. It is thought to improve acupoint stimulation and may be used to treat pain and other musculoskeletal disorders.

2. Acupressure: Instead of needles, acupoints are stimulated using pressure applied with the fingers, palms, or specialized instruments.

This method is frequently used for self-care and can help relieve stress and promote relaxation.

3. Moxibustion is the practice of burning dried mugwort (moxa) near or on acupoints to enhance Qi flow and facilitate healing. For particular illnesses, moxibustion is frequently used in combination with acupuncture.

4. Cupping: Suction is created by applying glass or plastic cups to the skin, boosting blood flow and reducing muscular tension. Cupping is frequently used to treat pain, inflammation, and respiratory issues.

5. Gua Sha: This treatment includes scratching the skin with a smooth-edged object to increase blood circulation and decrease inflammation. Gua sha is commonly used for musculoskeletal ailments and is thought to expel toxins from the body.

Acupuncture Types

Acupuncture methods and approaches have developed throughout time, reflecting geographical influences as well as individual preferences. Well-known acupuncture treatments include:

1. Traditional Chinese Acupuncture: This is the classical kind of acupuncture that resolves Qi and meridian imbalances based on TCM principles.

2. Japanese acupuncture is characterized by shallower needle insertion and a softer approach. For diagnosis, Japanese acupuncture may use probing of the belly and hara (abdominal region).

3. Korean Hand Acupuncture: This one-of-a-kind technique concentrates on acupoints on the hands, particularly the fingers. It is frequently utilized due to its ease of use and accessibility.

4. Auricular Acupuncture: This treatment stimulates acupoints on the ear, which mirror the entire body. It is frequently used in the treatment of addiction, pain management, and stress reduction.

5. Scalp Acupuncture: This specialized kind of acupuncture targets points on the scalp and is commonly utilized for neurological problems including stroke recovery.

Acupuncture, in conclusion, is a comprehensive and ancient therapeutic therapy that is profoundly anchored in the principles of Traditional Chinese Medicine. Acupuncture has a rich history that dates back thousands of years and continues to expand, using numerous techniques and styles to address a wide range of health conditions. Acupuncture seeks to enhance general well-being and assist the body's natural healing processes by stimulating acupoints and harmonizing the flow of Qi.

The wide range of acupuncture techniques and styles illustrates this ancient practice's flexibility to many cultural settings and individual demands, which contributes to its ongoing appeal and efficacy in improving health and vitality.

CHAPTER TWO

Acupuncture Needles And Supplies

Acupuncture, a vital component of traditional Chinese medicine, has grown in popularity across the world due to its holistic approach to health and well-being. The needles and equipment utilized in the therapeutic procedure are fundamental to this ancient discipline. Acupuncture needles, unlike hypodermic needles used in traditional medicine, are thin, sterile, and firm, and are meant to stimulate particular places on the body.

Acupuncture needles come in a variety of lengths and sizes, allowing practitioners to personalize treatments to the needs of the individual. Stainless steel is the most often used material for these needles, offering both durability and flexibility. Despite their thinness, these needles are incredibly strong, offering a pleasant and efficient method of delivering acupuncture's curative benefits.

The placement of needles into precise places known as acupuncture points or acupoints is essential to the effectiveness of the therapy. The accuracy and skill required in needle insertion have a substantial impact on therapeutic success. Acupuncture needles are often put just beneath the skin's surface, and the feeling is frequently characterized as tingling or a dull discomfort. The depth and angle of insertion are determined by the acupoint being targeted as well as the individual's condition.

Aside from needles, acupuncture therapy employs a variety of different methods. Moxibustion is the practice of burning mugwort herb near acupoints to promote healing and energy flow. Cupping, another complementary therapy, employs suction to increase blood circulation. Electroacupuncture employs the use of a small electric current to stimulate the needles. These additional procedures supplement the use of acupuncture needles, giving a comprehensive and tailored therapeutic strategy.

The Functions Of Acupuncture Points

The notion of qi, or vital energy that travels via meridians or channels in the body, is central to the theory of acupuncture. Acupuncture points, also known as acupoints or acupressure points, are precise sites along these meridians that may be reached and changed by qi. Each acupoint refers to a certain organ, system, or function of the body.

There are about 350 identified acupoints, and their choice is determined by the patient's diagnosis and intended treatment outcome. The stimulation of these sites is said to restore qi equilibrium, improve health, and treat a variety of diseases.

The functions and connections of acupuncture sites inside the body are used to classify them. Some points, for example, are classified as tonifying or strengthening, while others are classified as dispersing or diminishing.

The points are chosen to address the individual's particular constitution as well as the precise patterns of imbalance discovered during the diagnostic.

Understanding the activities of acupoints necessitates familiarity with traditional Chinese medical philosophy, which regards the body as a holistic organism with interconnected energy lines. Stimulating acupoints on the Liver meridian, for example, may address issues associated with liver disease, such as menstruation irregularities or emotional disorders.

Acupoint stimulation is normally accomplished by the insertion of acupuncture needles, while alternative modalities such as acupressure, laser treatment, or electroacupuncture can also be used. Practitioners want to restore equilibrium within the body and increase overall well-being by altering the flow of qi through these locations.

The Acupuncture Diagnosis Process

A comprehensive diagnostic is required before beginning acupuncture therapy to discover the underlying patterns of imbalance in the patient's body. Traditional Chinese medicine diagnosis takes a comprehensive approach, taking into account not just the symptoms but also the individual's constitution, lifestyle, and environmental circumstances.

Inspection, hearing and smelling, questioning, and palpation are the four basic examination procedures used in acupuncture diagnosis. Physical qualities such as the tongue, skin, and facial features are examined during inspection. Changes in tongue color, coating, and shape reveal important information about the patient's internal balance. Listening and smelling entails paying attention to the patient's speech, breath, and body odor, which might provide further information about the underlying imbalance.

Inquiry is a thorough interview procedure in which the practitioner learns about the patient's medical history, lifestyle, food, and emotional well-being. This assists in determining the fundamental causes of the symptoms and adjusting the treatment accordingly. Palpation is the process of feeling certain regions of the body, such as the pulse and various acupuncture sites, to assess qi quality and detect areas of stress or imbalance.

Acupuncture practitioners analyze the pulse at numerous places on the radial artery to determine pulse diagnosis. The pulse is evaluated for depth, rhythm, and strength, which correspond to distinct organ systems and patterns of imbalance.

Acupuncturists build a thorough picture of the patient's health and formulate a treatment plan targeted to address the fundamental causes of their symptoms by integrating information from different diagnostic approaches.

Acupuncture differs from many traditional medical techniques in that it strives not just to relieve symptoms but also to restore balance and harmony to the entire body.

The Conditions Listed Below Are Treated By Acupuncture:

Acupuncture is beneficial in treating a wide range of acute and chronic illnesses. While it is most usually linked with pain treatment, its therapeutic reach is far broader. Acupuncture is widely used to treat the following conditions:

1. Acupuncture is well-known for its effectiveness in treating numerous forms of pain, including chronic pain disorders such as back pain, arthritis, and migraines. Acupuncture regulates pain signals, reduces inflammation, and promotes the body's natural healing mechanisms by stimulating certain acupoints.

2. Stress and Anxiety: Acupuncture has been demonstrated to be effective in relieving stress and

anxiety by encouraging relaxation and harmonizing the nervous system.

 Acupuncture's soothing effects are related to its capacity to control neurotransmitters and stress hormones.

3. Digestive Disorders: Acupuncture can help people with digestive difficulties such as irritable bowel syndrome (IBS), indigestion, and gastritis. Acupuncture helps improve digestion and nutrition absorption by correcting digestive system abnormalities.

4. Acupuncture is often used to treat women's health difficulties such as menstruation abnormalities, reproductive troubles, and menopausal symptoms. The treatment tries to promote overall reproductive health by regulating hormone balance.

5. Respiratory disorders: Acupuncture can help with respiratory disorders such as asthma, allergies, and sinusitis.

Acupuncture improves respiratory health by improving lung function and decreasing inflammation.

6. Acupuncture has been demonstrated to be useful in the treatment of insomnia and other sleep problems. The therapy encourages relaxation, modulates sleep-wake cycles, and tackles underlying problems that contribute to sleep disruption.

7. Acupuncture is said to boost the immune system by stimulating the flow of qi and regulating the body's energies. This may aid in the prevention of recurring infections as well as the general immune function.

8. Acupuncture has been studied as a supplemental therapy for neurological disorders such as migraine headaches, neuropathy, and stroke recovery. While not a cure, acupuncture may help people with certain disorders manage their symptoms and improve their quality of life.

It is crucial to highlight that acupuncture is frequently used in conjunction with conventional medical treatments as a complementary therapy.

 It is suggested that you consult with a certified healthcare expert to identify the most appropriate and successful treatment strategy for your specific health requirements.

CHAPTER THREE

Acupuncture For Pain Relief:

Pain treatment is one of the most well-established uses of acupuncture. The success of acupuncture in pain relief stems from its capacity to modify the neurological system, manage inflammation, and increase the production of endorphins, the body's natural analgesics.

Acupuncture is widely used to treat a variety of pain conditions, including musculoskeletal pain, neuropathic pain, and headaches. Acupuncture has been demonstrated to be effective in treating conditions such as back pain, osteoarthritis, and migraines. The effectiveness of the therapy in pain management is not just based on the insertion of needles, but on a holistic strategy that addresses the underlying causes of pain.

The effects of acupuncture on pain are regarded to be multi-dimensional. Acupuncture regulates the passage of pain signals along the nerve system by stimulating certain acupoints. This can lead to a decrease in pain perception and an increase in pain tolerance. Acupuncture also contains anti-inflammatory properties, which aid in the relief of pain linked with inflammatory disorders.

Another way by which acupuncture exerts its analgesic benefits is the release of endorphins, the body's inherent pain-relieving compounds. Endorphins work on the neurological system to diminish pain perception and promote happiness. This natural pain modulation is one of the reasons why acupuncture is seen as a comprehensive pain treatment technique, treating both the physical and emotional elements of pain.

The acupoints used for pain treatment are chosen based on the nature and location of the pain. Acupoints along meridians connected with the diseased location, for example, or those recognized for their analgesic characteristics, may be targeted.

Electroacupuncture, which includes passing a low electric current via the acupuncture needles, is often used to provide further pain relief.

Because of its usefulness in pain treatment, acupuncture has been included in conventional healthcare for ailments such as persistent low back pain, osteoarthritis, and postoperative pain. While individual reactions to acupuncture vary, many patients report considerable pain reduction and general well-being benefits from this ancient therapeutic therapy.

Finally, acupuncture is a comprehensive and adaptable therapy that stimulates acupoints in the body using specific needles and equipment. The acupoints are chosen based on their functions within the context of traditional Chinese medicine, to restore balance and harmony to the body's energy flow. Acupuncture's diagnostic procedure is thorough, taking into account multiple examination methods to customize treatments to the individual's particular constitution and imbalances.

Acupuncture has been demonstrated to be useful in the treatment of a variety of illnesses, including pain management, stress management, digestive problems, women's health difficulties, respiratory ailments, sleep disorders, immune system support, and neurological disorders.

Its use in pain management is well-established, with acupuncture modulating the neurological system, controlling inflammation, and boosting endorphin release to reduce pain.

As acupuncture becomes more widely used in mainstream medicine, continued research and clinical trials lead to a better knowledge of its mechanics and uses.

Acupuncture's holistic approach makes it a viable alternative for those seeking natural and tailored answers to diverse health conditions, whether utilized as a main or supplemental therapy.

Traditional Chinese Medicine And Acupuncture For Holistic Health

Acupuncture, a crucial component of Traditional Chinese Medicine (TCM), has been performed for hundreds of years and is based on the notion that the vital energy, or Qi, of the body travels along meridians. These meridians are thought to be conduits via which the body's energy is balanced. Illness arises when there is an imbalance or obstruction in the movement of Qi, according to TCM principles. Acupuncture attempts to reestablish this equilibrium by putting small needles into precise sites along the meridians, therefore boosting the body's natural healing mechanisms.

TCM's underlying premise of holistic health stresses the interdependence of the body, mind, and spirit. Acupuncture is regarded as a comprehensive therapy since it treats not just the symptoms of a disease, but also the underlying imbalances that may be contributing to the sickness. TCM practitioners evaluate the patient's total well-being by taking into account elements like as lifestyle, nutrition, emotions, and environmental influences. Acupuncture promotes comprehensive health and wellness by treating the full individual.

Aside from its medical effects, acupuncture is said to improve mental and emotional well-being. TCM considers emotions to be essential to health, and acupuncture is supposed to assist in balancing emotional states by altering Qi flow. Following acupuncture sessions, many people experience lower stress, greater mood, and more mental clarity.

Furthermore, TCM emphasizes the significance of prevention in preserving overall health. Acupuncture may be used as a preventative strategy to keep the body in balance and harmony, helping to keep ailments at bay. Acupuncture sessions regularly may be advised to improve overall well-being and prevent imbalances from evolving into more significant health problems.

Acupuncture In The 21st Century

Acupuncture has received significant recognition in the modern healthcare environment in recent years, with a growing amount of evidence confirming its usefulness for a variety of illnesses.

Acupuncture has evolved to treat a wide range of current health conditions, despite its historical roots in ancient Chinese medicine.

One significant application is in the treatment of pain. Organizations like the World Health Organization (WHO) have acknowledged acupuncture for its effectiveness in treating illnesses such as chronic pain, migraines, and osteoarthritis. The mechanism underlying this pain alleviation is considered to entail the production of endorphins, the body's natural painkillers, as well as nervous system regulation.

Acupuncture is also utilized to address mental health problems. Acupuncture may help with illnesses including anxiety, sadness, and sleeplessness, according to research.

Acupuncture's holistic approach resonates with current understandings of the interconnection of mental and physical health.

Acupuncture has also discovered benefits in women's health. It is often used to treat menstruation abnormalities, reproductive difficulties, and menopausal symptoms. Acupuncture's integrative nature makes it a good supplement to traditional medical therapies in these areas.

Acupuncture has also acquired popularity in sports medicine. Athletes seek acupuncture for pain relief, injury healing, and performance enhancement. Acupuncture is a popular choice among athletes searching for non-invasive therapies due to its ability to target particular parts of the body and encourage natural recovery.

CHAPTER FOUR

Integration Of Acupuncture And Western Medicine

Acupuncture's incorporation into Western medicine is an increasing trend, reflecting the awareness of its therapeutic effects. While traditional Western medicine depends on medicines and surgery, acupuncture provides an alternative method that can improve overall patient care.

One area of integration is chronic pain treatment. Acupuncture is increasingly being advocated as part of a multimodal pain management strategy, including pharmaceuticals and physical therapy. This integration enables a more thorough and tailored therapy approach that addresses both pain symptoms and underlying causes.

Acupuncture is also used to address adverse symptoms associated with traditional cancer therapies, such as nausea, exhaustion, and discomfort.

Acupuncture has been shown in studies to improve the quality of life for cancer patients receiving chemotherapy or radiation therapy. Integrating acupuncture into cancer therapy reflects a larger change in modern medicine toward holistic and patient-centered methods.

Acupuncture is frequently used in reproductive medicine in conjunction with assisted reproductive technologies (ART) such as in vitro fertilization (IVF). Acupuncture may boost ART success rates by increasing blood flow to the reproductive organs, lowering stress, and promoting general reproductive health, according to research.

A growing corpus of scientific data confirming the efficacy of acupuncture is facilitating its incorporation into Western medicine. Acupuncture's processes are becoming more understood as research develops, making it simpler to incorporate acupuncture into evidence-based medical procedures.

Acupuncture's Risks And Benefits

While acupuncture is usually seen to be safe when conducted by experienced and competent practitioners, it is important to be aware of any hazards and safety concerns.

The potential for infection is a major worry. Acupuncturists must use sterile, single-use needles and follow stringent cleanliness measures to reduce this danger. To reduce the possibility of problems, patients should verify that their acupuncturist follows adequate infection control protocols.

Another factor to consider is the likelihood of bruising or bleeding at the site of insertion. This is normally minimal and resolves on its own, but those with bleeding problems or who use blood thinners should notify their acupuncturist to reduce the risk.

More significant adverse effects, such as organ harm or nerve damage, have been documented in rare situations. However, these occurrences are relatively rare and are frequently connected with untrained practitioners. Using a trained and certified acupuncturist lowers the likelihood of such consequences.

Before having acupuncture, anyone with specific health concerns, such as a weakened immune system or a history of seizures, should check with their doctor. Pregnant women should also notify their acupuncturist about their pregnancy, as certain acupuncture sites are not recommended during pregnancy.

It is vital to highlight that the safety of acupuncture is mostly dependent on the practitioner's ability and knowledge. Choosing a qualified and well-trained acupuncturist minimizes the chance of adverse occurrences greatly.

Acupuncture Research And Evidence

Acupuncture research has developed over the last several decades, leading to a growing body of data confirming its usefulness for a variety of diseases.

While several elements of the processes of acupuncture are still being studied, numerous major conclusions have emerged.

Numerous studies have shown that acupuncture is useful in alleviating chronic pain disorders such as osteoarthritis, lower back pain, and migraines. Endorphin release and pain pathway modification in the nervous system are thought to be fundamental to acupuncture's analgesic effects.

In the field of mental health, evidence suggests that acupuncture may be beneficial for illnesses such as anxiety and depression. Acupuncture is known to impact neurotransmitters and alter the stress response, perhaps contributing to its therapeutic advantages for mental health conditions.

The role of acupuncture in conception and reproductive health has also been investigated. Acupuncture may enhance results for women undergoing reproductive treatments such as IVF by increasing blood flow to the uterus, controlling hormones, and lowering stress, according to research.

Acupuncture research has focused on neurological diseases such as migraine headaches and post-stroke rehabilitation. While additional research is needed, preliminary data shows that acupuncture may provide advantages in these regions via processes such as increased blood flow and neuroplasticity.

The rising number of systematic reviews and meta-analyses that have assessed the accumulated data supports the incorporation of acupuncture into mainstream healthcare. Acupuncture is frequently concluded to be a safe and effective supplementary treatment for a variety of diseases in these evaluations.

Finally, acupuncture, which has its roots in Traditional Chinese Medicine, has grown into a flexible therapy with applications in holistic health, pain management, mental health, reproductive medicine, and other areas.

Its incorporation into Western medicine represents a larger movement toward a more comprehensive and patient-centered approach to healthcare. While acupuncture is usually seen to be safe, it is critical to select a skilled practitioner and be aware of any hazards. The expanding volume of data confirming the efficacy of acupuncture helps its adoption and inclusion into evidence-based medical procedures, paving the way for a more integrative and completes healthcare system.

Acupuncture Education And Certification

Acupuncture therapy, which is based on traditional Chinese medicine, has acquired considerable acceptance and acknowledgment in the complementary and alternative medicine area. As the demand for acupuncture services grows, the significance of adequate training and certification becomes even more important. Acupuncturists get extensive study and training to guarantee that this ancient healing technique is used safely and effectively.

Acupuncture training normally consists of a combination of classroom instruction, hands-on practice, and clinical experience. Educational programs vary in duration and complexity, but they always address essential ideas such as traditional Chinese medical philosophy, anatomy, physiology, and acupuncture point selection principles. Many programs also include hands-on instruction in needling, herbal medicine, and other complementary therapies.

Acupuncture practitioners in the United States must graduate from a recognized acupuncture school and pass the National Certification Commission for Acupuncture and Oriental Medicine (NCCAOM) license test. The NCCAOM accreditation is widely accepted as a mark of expertise in the industry. Acupuncturists must enroll in continuing education to keep current with changes in acupuncture research and practice to maintain certification.

The certification procedure guarantees that acupuncturists have a firm grasp of the theoretical underpinnings of acupuncture and can use their knowledge in a clinical environment. It also protects the public by ensuring that practitioners follow established safety and ethical standards.

Many acupuncturists pursue further training in specialty fields such as sports acupuncture, fertility acupuncture, or pain treatment in addition to formal study and licensure. This continual education enables practitioners to broaden their knowledge and provide specialized services to a wide spectrum of clientele.

In conclusion, acupuncture education and certification are critical components of the profession. They equip practitioners with the information and skills needed to administer safe and effective acupuncture treatments while upholding high professional standards.

CHAPTER FIVE

Acupuncture In Different Cultures

Acupuncture, which is profoundly established in Chinese culture and philosophy, is more than just a therapeutic practice; it represents a comprehensive approach to health and well-being. Understanding cultural perceptions of acupuncture is critical for grasping its role in traditional Chinese medicine and recognizing its assimilation into other global healthcare systems.

Health is considered as a harmonious balance of vital energy or "qi" flowing through meridians in the body in traditional Chinese medicine. Acupuncture seeks to restore this equilibrium by stimulating particular sites throughout the meridians, supporting the body's innate healing capacities.

Acupuncture's conceptual framework is shaped by cultural ideas and traditions, which influence its diagnostic procedures, treatment tactics, and even the selection of acupuncture sites.

In Chinese culture, the body is viewed as a microcosm of the natural world, and acupuncture is based on the yin and yang principles.

Health is regarded as a dynamic balance of these conflicting forces. Illness occurs when there is an imbalance. Acupuncture attempts to restore equilibrium by regulating qi flow and balancing yin and yang.

As acupuncture moved over the world, it faced a variety of cultural situations and attitudes. Acupuncture is frequently included as a supplementary therapy in traditional medical procedures in Western countries. The emphasis may shift away from the traditional Chinese conceptual framework and toward a more scientific understanding of acupuncture's physiological effects on the neurological and endocrine systems.

Acupuncture acceptability and use are also influenced by cultural perceptions. Acupuncture is firmly rooted in healthcare traditions in several countries and is widely acknowledged as a mainstream treatment alternative. Skepticism may arise in others owing to cultural differences or a lack of experience with traditional Chinese medicine.

Furthermore, cultural knowledge is essential in providing acupuncture therapy. Practitioners must be sensitive to their clients' cultural origins, modifying their communication and treatment techniques accordingly. Respecting cultural differences means that acupuncture is not only effective but also accessible and acceptable to people from all walks of life.

Finally, from its ancient roots in Chinese philosophy to its incorporation into global healthcare practices, cultural viewpoints affect the foundation of acupuncture. Understanding and appreciating cultural differences is essential for both practitioners and patients to create a comprehensive and inclusive approach to acupuncture therapy.

Acupuncture Case Studies

Acupuncture case studies give significant insights into the many uses and efficacy of this ancient therapeutic method. These real-world examples demonstrate the variety of diseases that acupuncture may treat and highlight its potential as a supplemental therapy in a variety of healthcare settings.

Acupuncture is commonly used for pain treatment. Acupuncture has been shown in case studies to be useful in treating chronic pain disorders such as lower back pain, osteoarthritis, and migraines. Acupuncture needle placement has been demonstrated to modify pain signals, decrease inflammation, and encourage the production of endorphins, the body's natural analgesics.

Acupuncture has also shown potential in the treatment of mental health problems. Case studies show its role in lowering anxiety, sadness, and stress symptoms.

Acupuncture's holistic approach, which acknowledges the interdependence of the body and mind, is consistent with the ideas of integrative mental health therapy.

Acupuncture has also been used in fertility therapy. Based on case studies, acupuncture may increase fertility by regulating hormone balance, decreasing stress, and boosting blood flow to the reproductive organs. Acupuncture, while not a stand-alone treatment, is frequently used in complete fertility treatment strategies.

Case studies in sports medicine demonstrate the advantages of acupuncture in addressing sports-related ailments and improving athletic performance. Acupuncture may aid in injury rehabilitation by reducing inflammation and increasing range of motion. Athletes frequently use acupuncture as a non-pharmacological pain management and general well-being treatment.

It is crucial to remember that case studies add to the growing amount of data showing the efficacy of acupuncture, but they are not conclusive proof. While there are numerous individual success stories, more thorough research, including randomized controlled trials, is required to confirm acupuncture's efficacy across a wide variety of illnesses.

Finally, case studies provide insight into the various uses of acupuncture, ranging from pain management to mental health and fertility. While these stories are intriguing, further study is needed to confirm and improve our understanding of acupuncture's therapeutic potential.

Acupuncture Therapy's Future Trends

Several themes are affecting the future landscape of this ancient medical therapy as acupuncture evolves. These developments indicate the continual integration and spread of acupuncture within varied healthcare systems, ranging from technical breakthroughs to shifting healthcare philosophies.

1. Acupuncture's integration with mainstream medicine is a prominent development. As proof of the usefulness of acupuncture accumulates, more healthcare organizations are adopting it into their treatment programs. Acupuncturists and traditional medical practitioners are increasingly working together to provide patients with a more comprehensive and holistic approach to healthcare.

2. Technological Advances: Technology will play an important part in the future of acupuncture therapy. Electroacupuncture equipment, laser acupuncture, and acupressure applications are developing as alternatives for stimulating acupuncture sites. These advancements aim to improve the precision, consistency, and accessibility of acupuncture treatments.

3. Individual Variability in Response to Acupuncture: The awareness of individual variability in response to acupuncture is driving the creation of tailored treatment procedures. Acupuncture treatments are more successful when

they are tailored to a patient's specific constitution, symptoms, and preferences. This tailored approach is consistent with the wider trend in healthcare toward precision medicine.

4. Research and Evidence-Based Practice: As acupuncture becomes more popular, there is a greater emphasis on rigorous research and evidence-based practice. More clinical trials are being conducted by researchers to better evaluate acupuncture's usefulness for a variety of illnesses. Acupuncture's inclusion in evidence-based guidelines increases its legitimacy in the larger healthcare community.

5. Teleacupuncture and Remote Monitoring: With the introduction of teleacupuncture services, the rise of telehealth has spread to acupuncture. Acupuncture consultations and instruction may now be provided to patients virtually, increasing access to this therapy. Wearable gadgets and monitoring tools also allow practitioners to remotely track patients' progress and change treatment regimens as needed.

6. Acupuncture education is developing to suit the demands of a changing healthcare context. Acupuncture training is becoming more prominent in integrative medical schools.

Acupuncturists may now access online materials, virtual simulations, and interactive learning platforms thanks to continuous improvements in educational technology.

7. Globalization of Acupuncture Practices: The globalization of acupuncture is encouraging cross-cultural contact and collaboration among practitioners worldwide. This knowledge exchange adds to a more complete understanding of acupuncture's uses and cultural variances. In the acupuncture community, international conferences, research partnerships, and shared resources are becoming more common.

8. Acupuncture is gradually being recognized and regulated by governments and regulatory agencies as a genuine healthcare practice. The standardization of

educational qualifications, licenses, and professional standards for acupuncturists is part of this trend. Increased recognition fosters public trust and allows for further incorporation into mainstream healthcare.

Finally, the future of acupuncture therapy will be defined by integration, technology developments, customized care, and a dedication to evidence-based practice. Acupuncture is becoming a more useful and adaptable component of modern healthcare, with the ability to assist a wide range of patients and ailments as a result of these trends.

Conclusion

Finally, acupuncture treatment has developed as a compelling and all-encompassing approach to health and well-being. This old method, rooted in traditional Chinese medicine, has gained greater recognition and acceptance in modern healthcare. Patients frequently report not only symptom improvement but also a profound sense of balance and vigor throughout therapy.

Acupuncture may enhance the release of endorphins, aiding natural pain management, and modulating different physiological processes, according to research. Acupuncture has shown potential in tackling larger concerns such as stress, anxiety, and sleeplessness, in addition to its usefulness in treating particular conditions such as chronic pain, migraines, and musculoskeletal disorders.

Furthermore, the customized character of acupuncture treatments emphasizes its flexibility for a wide range of health conditions. Practitioners adjust sessions to each patient's specific needs, resulting in a more personalized therapeutic experience. Acupuncture, as a supplementary therapy, blends effortlessly into standard medical techniques, improving total patient care.

As scientists continue to investigate the processes underlying acupuncture's benefits, a growing body of data supports its significance in fostering holistic well-being.

The collected experiences of people who have undergone acupuncture therapy lead to the conclusion that it provides a beneficial and diverse path to obtaining optimal health and harmony in both body and mind.

THE END

54